AF499297

Contents

Copycat Restaurant Recipes You Should Try Asap

Craving a bowl of Panera's Broccoli Cheddar Soup? How about some Chick-fil-A Nuggets? Guess what, you don't have to hop in the car and drive somewhere to enjoy some of your favorite dishes! Thanks to our list of copycat recipes, you can enjoy all of your favorite restaurant dishes—like Cheesecake Factory Cheesecake and wings from Buffalo Wild Wings—right at home.

Here's how to make your favorite restaurant dishes with copycat recipes.

Copycat IHOP Pancakes

Prepartion time

5 minutes

INGREDIENTS

FOR THE WHIPPED BUTTER

1/2 c. butter, softened

2 tbsp. whole milk

FOR THE PANCAKES

- 2 c. all-purpose flour
- 3 1/2 tbsp. granulated sugar
- 1 1/2 tsp. baking powder
- 1 1/2 tsp. baking soda
- 1 tsp. kosher salt

- 2 c. buttermilk
- 2 large eggs
- 3 tbsp. melted butter
- Maple syrup, for serving

Instructions

FOR THE WHIPPED BUTTER

1. In a medium bowl using a hand mixer or whisk, beat together butter and milk until mixture is fluffy and scoopable, 2 to 3 minutes.
2. Cover with plastic wrap and set aside

FOR THE PANCAKES

1. Preheat oven to 200º.

2. In a large bowl, whisk together flour, sugar, baking powder, baking soda, and salt.

3. Make a well in the center of the flour mixture and pour in buttermilk.

4. Add eggs over buttermilk and whisk until combined, then fold in melted butter until just combined. (Clumps are OK!)

5. Preheat a large nonstick skillet over medium-low heat until hot but not scorching, 2 to 3 minutes.

6. Using a measuring cup, ladle ½ cup batter into the center of the skillet and use the bottom of the measuring cup to smooth batter out into a uniform circle about 5½" wide.

7. Cook 2 to 3 minutes until sides start to lift from the pan and bubbles start to form on top.

8. Flip, then cook an additional 1 to 3 minutes, or until the other side is golden brown.

9. Transfer to a baking sheet and keep warm in oven until ready to serve.

10. Repeat with remaining batter.

11. Top pancakes with a scoop of whipped butter and drizzle with maple syrupe.

Applebee's Grilled Chicken Oriental Salad

Prepartion time

20 minutes

Ingredients

- 1 pound boneless skinless chicken breast 2 portions
- 2 tablespoons olive oil
- 1/2 teaspoon salt
- 1/4 teaspoon black pepper
- 1/2 cup sliced almonds
- 8 cups romaine lettuce
- 1/4 cup shredded carrots
- 1/2 cup crispy rice noodles
- 4 tablespoons Applebees Oriental Salad Dressing

Instructions

1. Heat the grill to medium, or heat a cast-iron skillet or grill pan over medium heat.

2. Place the chicken breasts between two sheets of plastic wrap and gently pound them to 3/8-inch thick.

3. Brush chicken breasts with olive oil and season them with salt and pepper.

4. Grill chicken breasts for 5 to 7 minutes on each side, until cooked through. Transfer to a plate to rest for 4 to 5 minutes before slicing.

5. Toast the almonds in a small dry skillet over medium heat. Watch them carefully—there is a fine line between toasted almonds and burnt almonds! Shake the pan gently. When you begin to smell the almonds, toast for a few seconds

more, then immediately place the almonds on a paper towel. Allow them to cool for a moment or two.

6. Assemble salads by first putting the lettuce in bowls or on plates, 3 to 4 cups per serving.

7. Sprinkle each with 2 tablespoons of carrots, 1/4 cup crispy rice noodles, and 1/4 cup toasted almonds.

8. Arrange the chicken on top.

9. Serve with Applebee's Oriental Salad Dressing.

Panda Express Orange Chicken

Prepartion time

30 minutes

Ingredients

FOR THE CHICKEN:

- 2 lb boneless skinless chicken thighs, cut into 1" pieces
- 1 egg
- 1 1/2 tsp salt
- 1 pinch black pepper
- 2 tbsp oil divided, plus more for frying
- 1/2 cup cornstarch
- 1/4 cup flour

FOR THE SAUCE:

- 1 tablespoon corn starch
- 2 tablespoons rice wine
- 1/4 cup water
- 1 teaspoon sesame oil
- 3 tablespoons soy sauce
- 10 tablespoons sugar
- 10 tablespoons white vinegar
- zest of 1 orange

TO FINISH:

- 1 1/2 tablespoons ginger root minced
- 2 teaspoons garlic minced

- 1/2 tsp hot red chili pepper crushed

Instructions

1. To make the sauce combine the 1 tablespoon cornstarch, rice wine, water, sesame oil, soy sauce, sugar, white vinegar and orange zest.

2. To coat the chicken add the egg, salt, pepper and 1 tablespoon oil into a bowl and whisk together in a large bowl.

3. In a separate bowl, add 1/2 cup corn starch and flour and mix well.

4. In a large frying pan or a wok, heat oil in a wok 375 degrees.

5. Dip chicken pieces in the egg mixture, then dredge in the flour mixture.

6. Fry the chicken for 3 to 4 minutes or until golden and crisp.

7. Transfer to a cooling rack and repeat with remaining chicken.

8. When you are done with the chicken, drain most of the oil from the pan (leave about a tablespoon).

9. Add the ginger, garlic and crushed red peppers, cooking for about 10 seconds.

10. Add the orange sauce and bring to boil.

11. Turn off the heat, and add cooked chicken and stir until well mixed.

Panda Express Beijing Beef

Prepartion time

40 minutes

Ingredients

- 1 pound flank steak
- 1 cup canola oil
- 4 cloves garlic minced
- 1 yellow onion sliced
- 1 pieces red bell pepper cut into 1"
- 1/4 cup cornstarch divided
- 1/4 teaspoon salt
- 3 egg whites beaten

- 1 teaspoon cornstarch
- 1/2 cup water
- 1/4 cup sugar
- 3 tablespoons ketchup
- 6 tablespoons Hoisin sauce
- 1 tablespoon low sodium soy sauce
- 2 teaspoons oyster sauce
- 4 teaspoons sweet chili sauce
- 1 teaspoons crushed red peppers
- 2 tablespoons apple cider vinegar

Instructions

1. Cut the flank steak against the grain into thin 1/4 inch slices.

2. In a medium sized bowl add the beef, egg, salt and 1 teaspoon cornstarch and let marinate for 30 minutes to an hour.

3. To make the Beijing Beef Sauce, in a small bowl whisk together the 1/2 cup water, 1/4 cup sugar, ketchup, hoisin, soy sauce, oyster sauce, sweet chili sauce, crushed red peppers and apple cider vinegar.

4. After the beef has finishing marinating add 2 tablespoons cornstarch to a bowl, add the marinated beef (discard the extra marinade).

5. Heat a small saucepan with the oil on medium-high (I use a small saucepan so that I can get a deep fry on this without using a lot of

oil. So I fry in small batches, if you don't mind using more oil, go for a bigger pot and you can fry these up much faster).

6. With the last two tablespoons of cornstarch toss the beef one last time and shake off any excess cornstarch.

7. Fry the slices, in batches, until golden brown (2-3 minutes).

8. Heat a large pan on high heat and use two tablespoons of the oil you just fried the beef in.

9. Add the onion and bell pepper and cook for 2-3 minutes, until it just starts caramelizing on the edges.

10. Add the garlic in and continue to cook a few more seconds until fragrant.

11. Remove the veggies and put them with the beef on a plate.

12. Add the Beijing Beef sauce to the large pan and cook on high until it thickens, about 3-5 minutes.

13. Add the beef and vegetables into the sauce and toss to combine.

14. Serve immediately.

Panda Express Kung Pao Chicken

Prepartion time

40 minutes

Ingredients

- 1 pound boneless skinless chicken breast , diced into 1/2-inch pieces
- 1/4 cup water
- 1/2 teaspoon salt
- 1/2 large egg
- 1/4 cup cornstarch
- 2 tablespoons vegetable oil
- 1 teaspoon cooking wine (I used white wine)
- 2 1/2 tablespoons soy sauce (I use Kikkoman Reduced Sodium)
- 1/3 cup water
- 2 1/2 tablespoons vegetable oil (divided use)
- 12 whole dry chili peppers , smaller than 3 inches; if longer, cut in half

- 1/4 cup diced green onion , white part only, in 1/2-inch pieces
- 1 teaspoon ground ginger
- 1 teaspoon ground garlic
- 1 teaspoon crushed red chili pepper
- 1/2 tablespoon cornstarch mixed with 1/2 tablespoon water
- 1 teaspoon sesame oil
- 2 ounces dry roasted peanuts
- 1 red bell pepper , cut into 3/4 inch cubes
- 1 large zucchini , cut into 3/4 inch cubes

Instructions

1. Combine the chicken, 1/4 cup water, 1/2 teaspoon salt, 1/2 egg, 1/4 cup cornstarch and 2 tablespoons of vegetable oil and refrigerate at least 1 hour.

2. In a small bowl add the wine, soy sauce and water and set aside.

3. Heat wok/skillet on high heat 10 seconds, you want that pan to be nice and hot!

4. Add 2 tablespoons vegetable oil.

5. Remove chicken from marinade and add to wok, cooking on high heat for 60 seconds.

6. Remove the chicken from the pan, add another 1/2 tablespoon of oil and the red bell pepper and zucchini.

7. Cook on high and cook for 1-2 minutes, until just caramelized and slightly cooked.

8. Remove vegetables and add the chili peppers.

9. Stir until they darken a bit, then add the green onions, peanuts, ginger, garlic, crushed red pepper, and sesame oil.

10. Stir for 2-3 seconds and immediately add the wine/soy/water mixture.

11. Bring it to a boil, then add the cornstarch and water mix and stir until it has thickened.

12. Add the chicken and vegetables back in, stir to combine.

13. To make my chicken more like Panda Express I actually cut the chicken into large cubes then pulsed it twice in the food processor

for just a 1/2 second each just to break it apart and give is the same unique look.

Chipotle Inspired Jalapeno Lime Corn Salad

Prepartion time

5 minutes

Ingredients

- 1 lb supersweet yellow corn
- 2 jalapenos , very finely chopped (de-veined and de-seeded)
- 1/2 cup finely diced red onion

- 1/4 cup chopped fresh cilantro
- juice of 1 lime
- juice of 1 small lemon
- 1 1/2 tsp kosher salt
- 1/4 tsp pepper

Instructions

1. Mix all the ingredients together and let sit for an hour to let the flavors meld together.

Chipotle Chicken Recipe (Copycat)

Prepartion time

30 minutes

Ingredients

- 3 chicken breasts , boneless skinless
- 1 teaspoon kosher salt
- 1/2 teaspoon coarse ground black pepper
- 2 teaspoons chipotle chili powder
- 1 teaspoon dried oregano
- 1 teaspoon cumin
- 1/4 cup distilled vinegar
- 4 cloves garlic , minced
- 6 tablespoons rice bran oil , divided (vegetable oil is ok)
- 1/4 cup water

Instructions

1. Pound the chicken to an even thickness, about a half inch thick.

2. Add all the ingredients together (save 2 tablespoons of oil) in a large ziplock bag (removing as much air as possible), mixing it well together after closing, and marinate for at least 6 hours.

3. Remove from marinade and add to a medium high heat grill and cook for 5-6 minutes on each side until cooked through then chop roughly.

4. Add chopped chicken and 2 tablespoons of oil to a large pan on medium high heat to crisp for 4-5 minutes, stirring occasionally.

Chick-fil-A Nuggets (Copycat)

Preparation time

45 minutes

Ingredients

- 2 large eggs
- 1 cup milk
- 1 pound chicken breasts cut into 1" chunks
- 3/4 cup flour
- 3/4 cup breadcrumbs
- 2 tablespoons powdered sugar
- 2 teaspoons Kosher salt

- 1/2 teaspoon white pepper
- 1/4 teaspoon chili powder
- 3 inches of peanut oil

Instructions

1. In a food processor, add the breadcrumbs and process until very fine.

2. In a large ziplock bag or a bowl add the chicken pieces, the milk and the eggs and combine. (I usually just close the bag and squish it together)

3. Put the chicken in the fridge for 15-20 minutes.

4. In a large dutch oven fill it 3 inches deep with peanut oil and heat to 365-375 degrees

(medium high heat until a piece dropped in immediately bubbles up but doesn’t burn quickly).

5. Put the breadcrumbs, flour, powdered sugar, Kosher salt, white pepper, chili powder in a bowl and whisk together.

6. Dredge the chicken pieces in the flour mixture and let dry for a few minutes.

7. Fry in batches (avoid crowding them) until golden brown (2-3 minutes) and remove to a sheet pan.

8. Don’t drain on paper towels, it’ll create steam and soften the nuggets.

Chick-fil-A Market Salad

Preparation time

25 minutes

Ingredients

- 2 chicken breasts
- 1 tablespoon extra virgin olive oil
- 1/4 teaspoon kosher salt
- 1/8 teaspoon coarse ground black pepper
- 1/8 teaspoon cayenne pepper
- 1/4 teaspoon paprika
- 16 cups spring mix salad chopped

- 1 cup blueberries
- 1 cup strawberries cut in half
- 1 granny smith apple chopped
- 1/2 cup blue cheese crumbled
- 1 cup roasted walnuts
- 1 cup cup granola
- 1 cup Zesty Apple Cider Vinaigrette recipe below

Instructions

1. Combine the chicken, olive oil, kosher salt, black pepper, cayenne and paprika.

2. Heat a large skillet on medium heat and cook the chicken for 5-8 minutes on each side until cooked through.

3. Let chicken cool while assembling salad.

4. Layer the romaine, iceberg, cabbage, carrots, blueberries, strawberries, apple, blue cheese, roasted walnuts and granola.

5. Slice the chicken as thinly as you possibly can (refrigerated cooked chicken is easiest) and top on salad with vinaigrette.

Louisiana Chicken Pasta (Cheesecake Factory Copycat)

Prepartion time

35 minutes

Ingredients

CAJUN CREAM SAUCE

- 1 teaspoon red pepper flakes
- 1 teaspoon cajun seasoning
- 1/2 teaspoon Kosher salt
- 1/4 teaspoon ground black pepper
- 2 cups heavy cream

- 1 cup chicken stock
- 1 tablespoon cornstarch
- 1 cup Parmesan Cheese shredded

CRISPY PARMESAN CHICKEN

- 4 chicken breasts butterflied
- 1/4 cup flour
- 1 cup breadcrumbs
- 1/2 cup parmesan cheese grated
- 1/2 teaspoon Kosher salt
- 1/4 teaspoon ground black pepper
- 2 eggs
- 4 tablespoons vegetable oil

PASTA

- 1 lb Farfalle pasta
- 2 tablespoons butter
- 1/2 yellow bell pepper sliced
- /2 red bell pepper sliced
- 1/2 red onion sliced
- 8 ounces crimini mushrooms sliced
- 1 tablespoon minced garlic
- 1/4 cup parsley for garnish (optional)

Instructions

1. Mix the Sauce ingredients together and set aside.

2. Set a large pot of water to boil and cook the pasta to a minute shy of what is listed on the box.

3. Drain but do not rinse.

4. Mix the flour, breadcrumbs, Parmesan cheese, Kosher salt and black pepper together in one bowl.

5. In a second bowl whisk the eggs.

6. Dredge each piece of chicken into the breadcrumb mixture, then into the eggs, and finally back into the breadcrumb mixture.*

7. Let chicken sit on a tray while you cook the vegetables.

8. Melt butter in cast iron skillet over medium heat and add the bell peppers, onion, garlic and mushrooms.

9. Cook for 3-5 minutes until just starting to brown but not break down.

10. Remove the vegetables from the pan.

11. Add the 1/4 cup oil and cook the chicken until crispy and golden brown, 3-5 minutes on each side.

12. Remove the chicken from the pan and drain the oil.

13. Add the pasta and vegetables to the pan with the sauce mixture.

14. Let thicken and stir for 3-5 minutes.

15. While the sauce is cooking slice up the chicken.

16. Serve the pasta with the sliced chicken on top and extra Parmesan as desired.

Taco Bell Burrito Supreme (Copycat)

Prepartion time

30 minutes

Ingredients

- 1 pound ground beef , (80/20)
- 4 cups water
- 1 recipe Taco Bell Seasoning

- 3 cups refried beans
- 6 burrito sized flour tortillas
- 1 cup Taco Bell Red Sauce
- 1/4 yellow onion , minced
- 1 cup lettuce
- 1 cup sour cream
- 1 cup cheddar cheese , finely shredded
- 1 vine tomato , diced

Instructions

1. Add ground beef to a large pot with the water.

2. Bring to a boil and using a potato masher, mash the ground beef until completely broken apart.

3. Cook for 10 minutes, then drain all but about 1 cup of the water.

4. Add in the Taco Bell Taco Seasoning mix and stir well.

5. Cook until the liquid is reduced.

6. Wrap tortillas in damp paper towels and microwave for 20 seconds on 50% power.

7. Top each tortilla with refried beans, ground beef, Taco Bell red sauce, onions, lettuce, sour cream, cheddar cheese and tomatoes.

8. Fold in the top and bottom and wrap tightly before serving.

Honey Walnut Shrimp

Prepartion time

40 minutes

INGREDIENTS

- 1 c. water
- 1 c. granulated sugar
- 1 c. walnuts
- 1 lb. shrimp, peeled and deveined
- Kosher salt
- Freshly ground black pepper
- 2 large eggs, beaten

- 1 c. cornstarch
- Vegetable oil for frying
- 1/4 c. mayonnaise
- 2 tbsp. honey
- 2 tbsp. heavy cream
- Cooked white rice, for serving
- Thinly sliced green onions, for garnish

Instructions

1. In a small saucepan over medium heat, combine water and sugar and bring to a boil.

2. Add walnuts and let boil for 2 minutes.

3. Using a slotted spoon, remove walnuts and let cool on a small baking sheet.

4. Pat shrimp dry with paper towels and season lightly with salt and pepper.

5. Place eggs in a shallow bowl and cornstarch in another shallow bowl.

6. Dip shrimp in eggs, then in cornstarch coating well.

7. In a large skillet over medium heat, heat 1″ of oil.

8. Add shrimp in batches and fry until golden, 3 to 4 minutes.

9. Remove with a slotted spoon and place on a paper towel lined plate.

10. In a medium bowl, whisk together mayonnaise, honey, and heavy cream.

11. Toss shrimp in sauce.

12. Serve over rice with candied walnuts and garnish with green onions.

Copycat Big Mac

Prepartion time

25 minutes

INGREDIENTS

FOR THE SAUCE

- 3 tbsp. mayonnaise
- 3 tbsp. shallots, finely diced
- 3 tbsp. dill pickles, finely diced
- 3 tbsp. tomato ketchup

- 1 tbsp. Dijon mustard
- 1/2 tsp. onion powder
- 1/2 tsp. garlic powder
- 1/2 tsp. sweet paprika
- 1 tsp. white wine vinegar

FOR THE BURGER

- 2 tbsp. vegetable oil
- 1 lb. ground beef
- Kosher salt
- Freshly ground black pepper
- 1/2 white onion, finely diced
- 8 seeded burger buns

- 1/4 head iceberg lettuce, finely shredded
- 2 large dill pickles, thinly sliced
- 4 slices American cheese

Instructions

1. Make the burger sauce: In a medium bowl, add all sauce ingredients and whisk until smooth.

2. Refrigerate and allow flavors to combine for 1 hour.

3. In a separate bowl, season beef with salt and pepper and form into 8 equal balls (2 ounces each).

4. Press into a 4 3/4" ring mould to form a thin patty.

5. Place diced onion into ice cold water.

6. In a large skillet over medium heat, lightly toast buns, then set aside.

7. Add oil to pan and fry patties in two batches, cooking for 2 minutes per side, until cooked.

8. On four of the patties, top with a slice of cheese for the final minute to allow it to melt a little.

9. To assemble the burgers, spread some burger sauce across the bottom bun.

10. Sprinkle over some of the onions and shredded lettuce then add one burger patty.

11. Top with a second bottom bun, more burger sauce, onions, lettuce, and pickles.

12. Finally, top with the second burger patty and bun top.

13. Serve with classic fries and a can of Coke, if desired.

Copycat Chipotle Chicken

Prepartion time

2 hours 35 minutes

INGREDIENTS

FOR THE CHICKEN

- 1/2 red onion, roughly chopped
- 2 cloves garlic
- 1 chipotle pepper in adobo sauce, plus 2 tbsp. sauce
- 3 tbsp. vegetable oil
- Juice of 1 lime
- 1 tsp. dried oregano
- 1/2 tsp. ground cumin
- Kosher salt
- Freshly ground black pepper
- 1 lb. boneless skinless chicken breasts

FOR THE BOWLS

- Cooked Rice
- Corn
- Black beans
- Guacamole
- Salsa
- Lime wedges

Instructions

1. In a food processor, blend onion, garlic, chipotle pepper and adobo sauce, oil, lime juice, oregano, and cumin until smooth.

2. Season with salt and pepper.

3. Add marinade and chicken to a large resealable plastic bag and rub all over to coat chicken.

4. Let marinate in the fridge at least 2 hours.

5. Bring chicken to room temperature and preheat grill to high.

6. Remove chicken from marinade and discard marinade.

7. Grill chicken until cooked through and internal temperature reads 165°, about 8 minutes per side.

8. Serve chicken over rice with desired toppings.

Mrs. Fields Chocolate Chip Cookies

Prepartion time

45 minutes

INGREDIENTS

- 2 3/4 c. all-purpose flour
- 1 tsp. baking soda
- 3/4 tsp. kosher salt
- 1 c. (2 sticks) butter, cold, cut into cubes
- 1 c. packed dark brown sugar
- 1/2 c. granulated sugar
- 2 large eggs
- 2 tsp. pure vanilla extract

- 2 c. chocolate chips

Instructions

1. Preheat oven to 350° and line two large baking sheets with parchment paper.

2. In a medium bowl, whisk together flour, baking soda, and salt.

3. In another large bowl, using a hand mixer, cream together butter and sugars until mixture resembles coarse sand.

4. Add eggs, one at a time, beating well after each.

5. Scrape down sides of bowl, add vanilla, and beat until combined.

6. Add dry ingredients and mix until just combined, then stir in chocolate chips.

7. Using a medium cookie scoop, scoop dough 2" apart onto prepared pans.

8. Bake until golden and edges are set, but middles are still soft, 13 to 15 minutes.

BBQ Chicken Pizza

Prepartion time

35 minutes

INGREDIENTS

- 1 lb. refrigerated pizza dough, divided into 2 pieces
- 2 c. cooked shredded chicken
- 3/4 c. barbecue sauce, divided
- 1 c. shredded mozzarella
- 1/4 medium red onion, thinly sliced
- 1/3 c. shredded gouda
- Pinch crushed red pepper flakes (optional)
- 2 tbsp. freshly chopped cilantro

Instructions

1. Preheat oven to 500°.

2. Line two large baking sheets with parchment paper and grease with cooking spray. In a

medium bowl, stir together chicken and 1/4 cup barbecue sauce.

3. On a lightly floured surface, roll out pizza dough into a large circle, then slide onto prepared baking sheet.

4. Top each pizza with 1/4 cup barbecue sauce, then half the chicken mixture, spreading in an even layer and leaving 1" around the edge bare.

5. Next add an even layer of mozzarella and red onion, then top with gouda.

6. Sprinkle with crushed red pepper flakes if using.

7. Bake until cheese is melty and dough is cooked through, 20 to 25 minutes.

8. Garnish with cilantro before serving.

Chai Latte

Prepartion time

35 minutes

INGREDIENTS

- 6 cardamom pods
- 2 cinnamon sticks
- 1 star anise
- 2 tsp. whole cloves
- 1 tsp. black peppercorns
- 1 (1") piece fresh ginger, thinly sliced
- 1/3 c. packed brown sugar

- 4 c. water
- 6 black tea bags
- 1 tsp. pure vanilla extract
- 4 c. whole milk
- Ground cinnamon, for garnish
- Ground cardamom, for garnish

Instructions

1. In a small pot over medium heat, bring spices, sugar, and water to a boil.
2. Reduce heat and let simmer for 5 minutes.
3. Bring mixture back to a boil, then add tea bags and vanilla and remove from heat.
4. Cover and let steep for 10 minutes.

5. Remove tea bags then strain tea and discard spices.

6. In a medium pot over medium heat, bring milk to a simmer.

7. Turn off heat and use an immersion blender to froth milk.

8. To each mug, pour 3/4 cup chai tea and ½ cup warm milk, adjusting amounts according to preference.

9. Top off each mug with milk foam and a sprinkle of ground cinnamon and cardamom.

Copycat Taco Bell Stackers

Prepartion time

35 minutes

INGREDIENTS

- 1 tbsp. extra-virgin olive oil
- 1 onion, chopped
- 2 cloves garlic, minced
- 1 lb. ground beef
- 2 tsp. chili powder
- 1 tsp. paprika
- 1/2 tsp. ground cumin
- Kosher salt
- Freshly ground black pepper
- 4 large flour tortillas

- 1 1/2 c. nacho cheese sauce
- 2 c. shredded cheddar

Instructions

1. In a large skillet over medium heat, heat oil.
2. Add onion and cook until soft, 5 minutes.
3. Add garlic and cook until fragrant.
4. Stir in ground beef, breaking up meat with a wooden spoon, and cook until no longer pink, about 6 minutes.
5. Drain fat.
6. Stir in spices and season with salt and pepper.

7. Spread a thin layer of nacho sauce over one side of each tortilla, then top with ground beef and cheddar.

8. Fold tortillas in half to make quesadillas.

9. Heat a large nonstick skillet over medium heat. Working one at a time, add quesadillas.

10. Cook until golden (but not too crispy!), about 2 minutes. Flip and immediately fold the tortilla into thirds.

11. Cook 2 minutes more per side. Repeat with remaining quesadillas.

Copycat Olive Garden Breadsticks

Prepartion time

1 hour

INGREDIENTS

- 1 1/2 c. warm water
- 1 (1/4 oz) package active dry yeast
- 4 c. flour, plus more for surface
- 2 tbsp. Butter, softened to room temperature
- 2 tbsp. sugar
- 1 tbsp. kosher salt, plus more for finishing
- 2 tbsp. butter, melted
- 1 tsp. garlic powder
- Marinara, for dipping

Instructions

1. In a large bowl, combine water with yeast and set aside until foamy, 4 to 5 minutes. Next, add the flour, butter, sugar, and salt.

2. Mix with a wooden spoon until all ingredients are fully incorporated and a dough has formed.

3. On a floured surface, knead the dough until smooth, about 3 to 5 minutes.

4. Place on a large parchment sized baking sheet and cover with a kitchen cloth.

5. Let rise for 45 minutes.

6. Meanwhile, preheat the oven to 400° and line a baking sheet with parchment paper.

7. Cut dough into 12 small balls. Knead and stretch each ball into a breadstick about 8" long and 1" wide.

8. Place on prepared baking sheet and let rest for 10 minutes.

9. Brush with butter and bake until golden, 20 minutes.

BBQ Chicken Skillet Pizza

Prepartion time

40 minutes

INGREDIENTS

- 1 tbsp. extra-virgin olive oil, plus more for brushing
- 1/2 lb. boneless skinless chicken breasts, cut into 1" pieces
- Kosher salt
- Freshly ground black pepper
- All-purpose flour, for dough
- 1 lb. pizza dough, at room temperature
- 2 tbsp. barbecue sauce, plus more for drizzling
- 1/2 c. shredded cheddar
- 1/2 c. shredded fontina
- 1/4 small red onion, thinly sliced

- Ranch dressing, for drizzling
- Freshly chopped chives, for garnish

Instructions

1. Preheat oven to 500°.

2. In a large skillet over medium-high heat, heat oil.

3. Add chicken and cook until golden and no longer pink, 6 minutes per side.

4. Season generously with salt and pepper.

5. Meanwhile, brush an ovenproof skillet with oil.

6. On a floured work surface, roll out dough until circumference matches your skillet. Transfer to skillet.

7. Leaving a 1/2" border for crust, spread barbecue sauce onto dough. Top with cheddar, fontina, chicken, and red onion.

8. Brush crust with olive oil and sprinkle with salt.

9. Bake until crust is crispy and cheese is melty, 23 to 25 minutes.

10. Drizzle with barbecue sauce and ranch and garnish with chives.

Smoked Mozzarella Fondue

Prepartion time

30 minutes

INGREDIENTS

- 8 oz. cream cheese, softened to room temperature
- 1 c. smoked mozzarella
- 1 c. provolone
- 1/2 c. freshly grated Parmesan
- 1/3 c. sour cream
- 1/2 tsp. dried thyme
- 1/2 tsp. Italian seasoning
- 1/4 tsp. red pepper flakes
- kosher salt
- Freshly ground black pepper

- 1 small tomato, chopped
- 1 tbsp. parsley, finely chopped

Instructions

1. Preheat oven to 350° F.
2. In a large bowl, combine cream cheese, cheeses, sour cream, thyme, Italian seasoning and red pepper flakes.
3. Stir together until smooth and fully combined.
4. Season with salt and pepper.
5. Transfer cheese mixture into a small skillet. Bake until cheese is bubbling, around 20-25 minutes.
6. Broil if desired.

7. Garnish with tomato and parsley and serve with baguette.

Garlic Rosemary Chicken

Prepartion time

1 hour 35 minutes

INGREDIENTS

- 1 tsp. plus 2 tbsp. extra-virgin olive oil, divided
- 1 head garlic, top sliced off
- 4 chicken breasts, pounded 1/2" thick
- kosher salt
- Freshly ground black pepper

- 4 oz. cremini mushrooms, sliced
- 2 tbsp. unsalted butter, divided
- 1/4 c. white wine
- 3/4 c. chicken broth
- 3 sprigs fresh rosemary
- 5 oz. baby spinach
- Juice of 1/2 a lemon
- Mashed potatoes, for serving

Instructions

1. Preheat oven to 400°.

2. Drizzle a teaspoon of olive oil over garlic and wrap in foil.

3. Bake until golden and soft, about an hour.

4. Set aside to cool, then pick out cloves. Set aside.

5. In a large skillet over medium-high heat, heat remaining 2 tablespoons oil.

6. Season chicken breasts with salt and pepper, then sear until golden, about 8 minutes per side.

7. Transfer to a plate.

8. Return skillet to medium heat, add more oil if necessary, then add mushrooms.

9. Season with salt and pepper and cook until slightly wilted, 5 minutes.

10. Add butter and let melt, then stir in the garlic cloves, white wine, chicken broth, and rosemary.

11. Bring to a simmer, nestle back in chicken, and let simmer until sauce has reduced slightly, 6 to 7 minutes.

12. Stir in spinach and lemon juice and let cook until spinach is slightly wilted, about 2 minutes more.

13. Serve with mashed potatoes.

Tonga Toast

Prepartion time

30 minutes

INGREDIENTS

FOR THE STRAWBERRY COMPOTE

- 1 1/2 c. chopped strawberries
- 3 tbsp. sugar
- 1 tbsp. lemon juice
- 1 tsp. pure vanilla extract
- FOR THE TOAST
- 1 loaf white bread, unsliced
- 2 Bananas, sliced
- 4 large eggs
- 1 c. heavy cream
- 1 tbsp. sugar
- 1 tsp. cinnamon
- 1 tsp. pure vanilla extract
- Vegetable oil, for frying

- 1 c. cinnamon sugar
- sliced strawberries, for serving
- Maple syrup, for serving

Instructions

1. Make strawberry compote: In a small skillet over medium heat, combine strawberries, sugar, lemon juice and vanilla.

2. Bring mixture to a simmer and cook until the strawberries begin to break down and the mixture has thickened slightly, about 5 minutes.

3. Remove from heat and gently mash the compote with the back of a fork (or a potato masher).

4. Slice bread into 3 to 4 very thick pieces.

5. Use a knife to create a slit in one side of the toast, then stuff banana slices into the toast.

6. Repeat with remaining bread pieces and bananas.

7. In a medium bowl, whisk together eggs, milk, sugar, cinnamon and vanilla.

8. Dunk each stuffed sliced into the batter mixture, tossing to coat all sides.

9. Pour a 1/4" of vegetable oil into skillet and heat over medium heat.

10. When the oil is hot, add the battered bread and cook until crispy and golden all over, about 2 minutes per side.

11. Drain toast briefly on a wire rack.

12. Pour cinnamon sugar into a large shallow bowl, then gently shake off excess oil from warm toast and toss in cinnamon sugar.

13. Garnish with fresh strawberries and serve with strawberry compote and maple syrup.

Texas Cinnamon Butter

Prepartion time

10 minutes

INGREDIENTS

- 2 sticks (1 cup) butter, softened
- 1/4 c. honey
- 1 tsp. ground cinnamon, plus more for sprinkling
- 1 tsp. kosher salt
- 1/2 tsp. pure vanilla extract

Instructions

1. In a large bowl, combine all ingredients.
2. Using a hand mixer, beat all ingredients until fully combined and butter is slightly whipped.
3. Place butter in a ramekin and garnish with a sprinkle of cinnamon.

4. Slather on everything.

Chicken Bake

Prepartion time

1 hour

INGREDIENTS

- 1/2 lb. bacon
- 2 tbsp. extra-virgin olive oil, divided
- 1 lb. chicken breast
- 1 tsp. Italian seasoning
- kosher salt
- Freshly ground black pepper

- 1/2 c. freshly grated Parmesan, plus more for sprinkling
- 1 lb. pizza dough
- 1/4 c. Caesar dressing
- 2 c. shredded mozzarella, plus more for sprinkling
- 2 green onions, thinly sliced
- Egg wash
- 2 tbsp. chopped parsley

Instructions

1. Preheat oven to 425° and line a baking sheet with parchment paper.

2. In a large skillet over medium heat, cook bacon until crispy.

3. Drain on a paper towel-lined plate then chop into small pieces.

4. Wipe skillet clean.

5. To the same skillet, heat olive oil over medium-high heat.

6. Season both sides of chicken breasts with Italian seasoning, salt and pepper.

7. Add chicken to skillet and cook until golden on both sides, 6 to 8 minutes.

8. Remove from skillet and let rest for 5 minutes before chopping into small pieces.

9. Divide pizza dough into two pieces.

10. On a lightly floured surface, roll and stretch pizza dough to about 1/4" thickness.

11. Spread half the Caesar dressing onto pizza dough and top with half of each the chicken, bacon, mozzarella, Parmesan, and green onions.

12. Roll the pizza dough into a large log.

13. Repeat with remaining ingredients.

14. Transfer logs to the prepared baking sheet.

15. Brush with egg wash and sprinkle with more cheese and Italian seasoning.

16. Bake until golden and the dough is cooked through, about 25 minutes.

17. Garnish with parsley, then slice and serve warm.

Cilantro Lime Rice

Prepartion time

30 minutes

INGREDIENTS

- 1 tbsp. butter
- Juice of 2 limes, divided
- 1/2 tsp. kosher salt
- 1 c. basmati rice
- 2 c. water
- 1 tbsp. freshly chopped cilantro

Instructions

1. In a large saucepan over low heat, melt butter.

2. Add juice from one lime, salt and rice, stirring for one minute to coat.

3. Add water and bring to a boil.

4. Once boiling, cover and reduce to a simmer, cooking over low heat until rice is tender, 22 to 25 minutes.

5. Fold in cilantro, garnish with more lime juice and serve.

Strawberry Dressing

Prepartion time

30 minutes

INGREDIENTS

FOR THE DRESSING

- 1/2 c. strawberries, hulled and halved
- 3 tbsp. apple cider vinegar
- 1 tbsp. honey
- 1/3 c. extra-virgin olive oil
- 1/4 tsp. poppy seeds

FOR THE SALAD

- 8 oz. baby spinach
- 1 c. strawberries, hulled and sliced
- 1/3 c. crumbled feta
- 1/3 c. sliced, toasted almonds

Instructions

1. Make dressing: To a food processor, add strawberries, vinegar, and honey and blend until smooth.

2. Pour in olive oil and blend until emulsified.

3. Add poppy seeds and blend 1 second more.

4. To a serving bowl, add spinach, sliced strawberries, feta, and toasted almonds.

5. Toss with dressing and serve immediately.

Copycat Cracker Barrel Pancake

MAKES 5 SERVINGS

INGREDIENTS

1 cup all-purpose flour

3/4 teaspoon baking powder

1/2 teaspoon baking soda

1/2 teaspoon salt

1 cup buttermilk

1 egg

2 tablespoons butter, melted Extra butter, for the griddle Pure maple syrup

HOW TO MAKE IT

1. Mix the flour, baking powder, baking soda, and salt in a large bowl together. I recommend

using an electric mixer if you have one (I love my KitchenAid!)

2. In a smaller bowl, whisk an egg. Add in the buttermilk and the melted butter.

3. Mix in buttermilk egg mixture with dry ingredients until the batter is smooth

4. Run a stick of butter over a warmed griddle (or a large, flat frying pan.) Be careful, you don't want it too hot! This will scorch the pancakes...and your hands.

5. For larger pancakes similar to Cracker Barrel's, pour on a 1/2 cup batter for each pancake (makes about 5)

6. For smaller pancakes, pour on a 1/4 cup batter for each pancake (makes about 10)

7. Serve with Cracker Barrel maple syrup and butter.

Copycat Wendy's Chili

MAKES 8 SERVINGS

INGREDIENTS

1 garlic clove, minced

1 tablespoon olive oil

1 medium onion, diced

2 celery stalks, diced

1 green bell pepper, diced

1 lb. ground beef

1 tablespoon taco seasoning

1 10 oz can. pinto beans

1 10 oz. can kidney beans

1 10 oz. can tomato sauce

1 10 oz. can diced tomatoes

Shredded cheddar cheese, for topping

Sour cream, for topping

HOW TO MAKE IT

1. Heat up a dutch oven or a stockpot over medium heat. Add in the olive oil, minced garlic, onion, celery, and green bell pepper. When the vegetables start to become soft (about three minutes), add in the ground beef.

2. Using a wooden spoon, break up the ground beef and stir in with the vegetables. When the ground beef is no longer pink, using a spoon, drain the grease into an excess can.

3. Add in the beans, tomato sauce, and diced tomatoes into the dutch oven. Sprinkle in the taco seasoning and mix together.

4. Turn the chili on simmer, and let it cook for at least 30 minutes, stirring once in a while so nothing burns at the bottom. The longer you let it sit, the better the flavors will become.

5. Serve with shredded cheese and sour cream, if desired.

Copycat Shake Shack Sauce

MAKES 4 SERVINGS

INGREDIENTS

Shake Shack Sauce

1/2 cup mayo

1 tbsp ketchup

1/4 tsp cayenne pepper

1 teaspoon yellow mustard

1 tbsp dill pickle brine

Shake Shack Burger

1 lb ground beef

8 lettuce leaves

8 tomato slices

4 hamburger potato buns

4 slices American cheese

1 tablespoon butter

Salt & pepper

HOW TO MAKE IT

1. To make the sauce, whisk all of the ingredients together in a bowl.

2. For the burger, split the ground beef evenly into 4 oz. portions (this should make 4 patties).

3. Form them into a burger patty with your hands. Press down on them so the patties are thin—they will shrink when cooking.

4. Season each side of the patty with salt and pepper.

5. Heat up a cast-iron skillet over medium heat. Once hot, melt the butter in the skillet.

6. Throw the patties on the skillet. Cook on each side for 5 minutes.

7. When you flip the patties to the other side, press them down with a metal spatula, then add the slice of cheese.

8. While the patties are cooking, slice up the veggies. Spread some sauce on both sides of the bun.

9. For the proper copycat Shake Shack burger, add the patty with cheese to the bottom of the bun. Place 2 tomato slices and 2 lettuce leaves.

10. Serve with crinkle-cut fries

Copycat Cheesecake Factory Cheesecake

MAKES 10 SERVINGS

INGREDIENTS

For the cheesecake

8 oz. cream cheese, at room temperature

8 oz. sour cream

1 cup sugar

1 tsp vanilla extract

3 eggs

1 1/2 cups water

Fresh berries, for topping

For the crust

10 graham crackers

5 tbsp butter, melted

HOW TO MAKE IT

1. Preheat the oven to 350 degrees.

2. Place the graham crackers in a large plastic bag and seal. Using a rolling pin, roll over the graham crackers until they are crushed to a sand-like consistency.

3. Mix the crushed graham crackers with the melted butter in a bowl. Press into a springform pan.

4. Prebake the crust for 10 minutes. Set it out to cool.

5. While the crust is cooling, whisk the cream cheese and sugar together using an electric mixer.

6. Once the sugar is worked through the cream cheese, add the sour cream and vanilla extract. Add in the eggs next, one at a time.

7. When the eggs are worked into the cheesecake mixture, stop mixing. You do not want to overmix or the cheesecake will crack in the oven.

8. Heat up the water in a kettle or a pot over the stove, or even in the microwave until the water is hot.

9. Wrap the bottom of the springform pan in aluminum foil, then place it on a sheet pan with rimmed edges.

10. Pour the cheesecake mixture into the springform pan with the crust.

11. Carefully pour the hot water into the sheet pan, creating a water bath around the cheesecake.

12. Place the sheet pan (with the cheesecake on it) in the oven.

13. Bake for 55 minutes. The cheesecake will be slightly wobbly in the middle, that's okay.

14. Open up the oven door slightly and let it sit for 1 hour to cool.

15. Let the cheesecake refrigerate for 3-4 hours, or overnight.

16. Loosen the rim of the cheesecake from the pan using a spatula or a knife. Open up the springform pan.

17. Serve with fresh berries, whipped cream, chocolate sauce, or any other desired toppings!

Copycat Cracker Barrel Hashbrown Casserole

MAKES 12 SERVINGS

INGREDIENTS

- 1 bag frozen hashbrowns (about 2 lbs.)
- 1/2 medium onion, diced
- 1 stick butter, melted (1/2 cup)
- 1 10 oz. can cream of chicken
- 16 oz. sour cream
- 2 cups shredded cheddar cheese
- Cooking spray
- Bacon, optional
- Colby jack slices, optional

HOW TO MAKE IT

1. Preheat the oven to 375 degrees.

2. Mix together the frozen hashbrowns, onion, melted butter, cream of chicken, sour cream, and shredded cheddar cheese in a large bowl.

3. Spray down a deep casserole dish with cooking spray. Dump the hashbrown mixture into the pan.

4. Spread evenly in pan with a rubber spatula.

5. Bake in the oven for 45-60 minutes, or until the top is golden brown and the edges start to crisp.

6. Want a loaded hashbrown casserole? Melt slices of Colby jack cheese on top and sprinkle on some bacon. If you want the whole casserole to be loaded, add slices of cheese on top of the casserole during the last 10 minutes of cooking.

Copycat Red Lobster Biscuit

MAKES 8 SERVINGS

INGREDIENTS

- 2 cups all-purpose flour
- 1 Tbsp baking powder
- 1/2 tsp salt
- 1 tsp garlic powder
- 1 Tbsp chopped parsley
- 1/4 cup butter, cold
- 2/3 cup buttermilk
- 1/2 cup shredded cheddar cheese

HOW TO MAKE IT

1. Preheat the oven to 450 degrees.

2. Mix together the flour, baking powder, salt, and garlic powder in a large bowl.

3. Cut the butter into small cubes and work the cubes into the flour mixture.

4. Pour in the buttermilk and mix. Add cheddar cheese, then continue to mix.

5. Spray down a baking sheet. Scoop 1/4 cup of batter, shape into a biscuit with your hands, and place onto the sheet pan.

6. Bake for 10 minutes.

Copycat Panera Broccoli Cheddar Soup

MAKES 4 SERVINGS

INGREDIENTS

- 1/4 cup butter
- 1 onion, diced

- 1 garlic clove, minced
- 2 Tbsp all-purpose flour
- 2 carrots, shaved
- 2 cups chicken broth (or vegetable)
- 2 cups half and half
- 1 8 oz. block sharp cheddar cheese, shredded
- 2 broccoli crowns, broken into florets
- 1/2 tsp salt
- 1/4 tsp pepper

HOW TO MAKE IT

1. Heat a dutch oven (or a large pot) over medium heat. Melt in 1 tablespoon of the butter, then add in the diced onion and minced garlic. Sprinkle in the salt and pepper. Cook for 3 minutes.

2. Melt in the rest of the butter. Sprinkle in the flour and stir the onions until the flour is completely mixed in.

3. Pour in the broth. Slowly pour in the half in half while continuously whisking.

4. Add in the broccoli florets and the shaved carrots.

5. Cover the dutch oven and cook on low for 12 minutes, stirring occasionally.

6. Remove half of the soup to a blender. Blend until smooth.

7. Add the blended soup back to the dutch oven and stir in the shredded cheddar. Once the cheese has melted, serve.

Copycat Cracker Barrel Mac and Cheese

MAKES 6 SERVINGS

INGREDIENTS

- 1/3 cup butter
- 1/3 cup flour
- 2 cups dry macaroni
- 2 1/2 cups Colby cheese, shredded
- 2 cups milk
- 1 tsp salt

HOW TO MAKE IT

1. Boil water in a large pot, then cook the 2 cups of dry macaroni. Drain.

2. Turn on the broiler.

3. Heat a cast-iron skillet over medium-low heat. Once hot, add the butter.

4. When the butter is fully melted, sprinkle in the flour. Whisk together until the ingredients are fully mixed.

5. While whisking, slowly pour in the milk. Do a small amount at a time while whisking. The mixture will get super thick at first. As you continue to slowly pour all the milk in, it will become a creamy white sauce.

6. Sprinkle in 2 cups of the Colby cheese, and whisk together until the cheese is fully melted. Turn off the heat.

7. Mix in the cooked macaroni. Spread the macaroni and cheese evenly in the cast-iron skillet.

8. Sprinkle the last 1/2 cup of Colby cheese on top.

9. Place the cast-iron skillet in the broiler for 5 minutes.

Copycat Carrabba's Blackberry Sangria

MAKES 8-10 SERVINGS

INGREDIENTS

1/4 cup simple syrup

- 1 nip of brandy (about 1/4-1/3 cup)
- 1 cup cranberry juice
- 1 bottle of dry Spanish red wine
- 1 lemon, sliced
- 1 orange, sliced
- 1 cup blackberries

- 1 cup blackberries, crushed
- 1/2 tsp vanilla flavoring

HOW TO MAKE IT

1. In a bowl, crush 1 cup of blackberries. Remove the soft pits out of the bowl and compost them (or eat them!)

2. Place the lemon slices, orange slices, whole blackberries, and crushed blackberries into the pitcher.

3. Pour in the simple syrup, the brandy, and the cranberry juice.

4. Add in the whole bottle of red wine.

5. Mix together with the vanilla flavoring. Vanilla extract will also work fine for this.

6. Chill in the refrigerator for 2 hours.

7. Serve over ice.

Copycat Shamrock Shake

MAKES 1 SERVING

INGREDIENTS

- 2 scoops vanilla ice cream
- 1/2 cup milk
- 1 drop peppermint extract
- 2 drops green food dye

HOW TO MAKE IT

1. Add in the scoops of ice cream to a blender, then pour in the milk.

2. Drop the extract and food dye into the blender.

3. Cover and blend for 15 to 20 seconds.

4. For a thicker shake, add more ice cream. For a thinner shake, add more milk.

5. Serve with whipped cream.

Copycat Carrabba's Chicken Marsala

MAKES 4 SERVINGS

INGREDIENTS

- 1 tbsp olive oil
- 2 tbsp butter, separated
- 4 chicken breasts
- 10 oz. sliced mushrooms
- 1 garlic clove, minced
- 1/2 onion, finely chopped
- 1/2 cup Marsala cooking wine
- 1/2 cup chicken stock
- 1/2 cup heavy cream

- 1 teaspoon cornstarch
- 1 tablespoon water
- 2 cups broccoli
- Salt and pepper

HOW TO MAKE IT

1. Bring a skillet to medium heat. Once the skillet is heated, melt 1 tablespoon of butter on the skillet.

2. Season both sides of each chicken breast with salt and pepper. Sear them on the skillet until the outside has started to brown, about 2-3 minutes each side. Remove to a separate plate.

3. In the same skillet, add the olive oil and the other tablespoon of butter.

4. Add the minced garlic and cook until fragrant, about 30 seconds.

5. Throw in the mushrooms, and cook for about 5 minutes.

6. While the mushrooms are cooking, boil some water in a large pot. Cook the broccoli for 5 minutes in the boiling water, then strain.

7. Slowly pour in the Marsala cooking wine, the chicken stock, then the heavy cream.

8. In a small bowl, mix together the cornstarch and the water to make a small slurry. Pour into the skillet.

9. Add in the chicken breast to the sauce, making sure each breast is covered with some of the sauce in the skillet.

10. Simmer for 10 minutes, or until the chicken is fully cooked (no longer pink on the inside) and the sauce has thickened.

11. Serve with the boiled broccoli.

Crispiest Oven-Fried Chicken

SERVES 4

INGREDIENTS

- 8 chicken drumsticks
- 4 cups non-fat buttermilk
- 1/4 cup salt
- 1/4 cup sugar
- 1 Tbsp hot sauce (preferably Frank's RedHot pepper sauce)
- 2 cups panko bread crumbs
- 2 Tbsp canola or vegetable oil
- 1 tsp chili powder
- 1/2 tsp garlic salt

HOW TO MAKE IT

1. Combine the chicken, buttermilk, salt, sugar, and hot sauce in a sealable plastic bag and shake to combine. Refrigerate for at least 2 hours or up to 12 hours.

2. Preheat the oven to 350°F.

3. In a large mixing bowl, use your fingers to break up the panko bread crumbs into slightly smaller pieces (this will help create a more even coating on the chicken).

4. Add the oil, chili powder, and garlic salt and stir to combine.

5. Working with one piece at a time, remove the chicken from the marinade, shake off the excess liquid, then toss in the bread crumbs until thoroughly coated.

6. Place the chicken pieces on a rack set in a rimmed non-stick baking sheet.

7. Bake on the middle rack of the oven for about 30 minutes, until the bread crumbs are evenly browned and the chicken is cooked through.

Old-Fashioned Milkshake

MAKES 1 SERVING

INGREDIENTS

For the milkshake

- 2 scoops french vanilla ice cream
- 1/2 cup milk
- For the flavor, pick one
- 1 Tbsp chocolate syrup
- 4 frozen strawberries

- 1 Tbsp peanut butter

HOW TO MAKE IT

Scoop in the ice cream

Scoop in two scoops of French Vanilla ice cream into a blender.

Pour in the milk

Pour in half a cup of milk. If you want a thicker consistency, use more ice cream and less milk.

Add your flavor

Add in whichever flavor you desire. For a chocolate milkshake, I add in about 1 tablespoon of chocolate syrup. The same goes for peanut butter. For a strawberry milkshake, blend up 4 frozen strawberries.

Blend for 10 seconds

Blend for 10 seconds, or until smooth, on low if possible. If the milkshake is too thick, add more milk. Too thin? Add in more ice cream.

Add toppings, if desired

Top your milkshakes with whatever toppings you desire. Traditionally, milkshakes are served with whipped cream and a cherry. But honestly, you can top them with sprinkles, chocolate—anything, really. The choice is yours!

FULL MILKSHAKE RECIPE

1. Add the scoops of ice cream to the blender. Pour in the milk.

2. For a flavored milkshake, add in the chocolate syrup (or whichever flavoring you desire).

3. Blend until smooth. If the consistency is too thick, add in a small amount of milk at a time until the shake thickness is to your liking. If too thin, add more ice cream.

4. Serve with whipped cream and toppings.

Copycat Egg Sandwich With Pastrami and Swiss

SERVES 4

YOU'LL NEED

- 1/2 Tbsp butter
- 4 oz lean pastrami (or turkey pastrami), cut into strips
- 6 eggs
- 2 Tbsp milk
- Salt and black pepper to taste

- 4 slices low-fat Swiss cheese
- 4 whole-wheat English muffins, lightly toasted

HOW TO MAKE IT

1. Melt the butter in a large nonstick skillet over medium heat. Add the pastrami and sauté for 2 to 3 minutes. Turn the heat down to low. Combine the eggs with the milk and a few pinches of salt and pepper. Whisk lightly, then add to the pan. Use a wooden spoon to constantly stir the eggs, scraping from the bottom as they set, as they'll continue to cook once removed from the stovetop.

2. Place a slice of Swiss on the bottom of each English muffin. Divide the scrambled eggs

among the muffins, top with the muffin tops, and serve.

Copycat Chipotle Pico de Gallo

MAKES ABOUT 3 CUPS

YOU'LL NEED

- 4 Roma tomatoes, chopped
- 1 small red onion, diced
- 1 jalapeño, minced
- 1 handful cilantro, chopped
- Juice of 1 lime
- Salt and pepper to taste

HOW TO MAKE IT

Combine the tomatoes, onion, jalapeño, cilantro, and lime juice in a mixing bowl. Season with salt and pepper and mix to thoroughly combine.

Keeps covered in the refrigerator for up to 1 week.

Copycat Starbucks Caramel Frappuccino

What You Need

- 1 cup strong brewed coffee, cooled
- 1 cup ice cubes
- 1 cup 1% milk
- ¼ cup low-fat vanilla frozen yogurt
- 1 Tbsp sugarfree caramel syrup
- ½ Tbsp agave syruppple cider caramel popcorn Recipe

How to Make It

Place all the ingredients in a blender and blend until smooth and uniform.

Mix It Up

Three ways to amp up the flavor:

Chocolate: Replace the caramel with a tablespoon of chocolate sauce (the darker the better) and a pinch of cinnamon.

Banana: Drop a frozen banana into the blender. Continue with the recipe.

Booze: Add a shot of Kahlua or Bailey's to any of the versions above.

Copycat Chick-fil-A Nuggets

MAKES 4 SERVINGS

INGREDIENTS

For the popcorn chicken:

- 1 lb boneless skinless chicken breasts, cut into 1 1/2-inch cubes
- 1 tsp chili powder
- 1 1/2 cups buttermilk
- 4 cups Arrowhead Mills Organic Spelt Flakes cereal
- 1/2 cup Bob's Red Mill Almond Flour
- 1/2 cup almond slivers
- Chosen Foods olive oil spray
- Freshly ground black pepper

Salt

For the chipotle aioli:

- 1/2 cup mayonnaise
- Juice of 1/2 lemon
- 1 tsp tomato paste
- 1/8 tsp salt

- 1/8 tsp garlic powder
- 1/4 tsp chipotle powder

HOW TO MAKE IT

1. Preheat oven to 425°F. Place a wire cooling rack over a baking sheet.

2. Season the chicken with chili powder and place in a large bowl. Pour the buttermilk over the chicken, cover the bowl, and marinate in the fridge for 2 hours.

3. To prepare the breading, combine the spelt cereal, almond flour, and almonds in a food processor. Pulse until you get a coarse meal with some larger flakes of cereal. Place in a bowl.

4. Remove the chicken from the marinade, and press each piece into the breading on all sides. Place on the rack and spray with oil.

5. Bake for 15 minutes, until the chicken is golden brown and reaches an internal temperature of 165°F. Remove from the oven and season the chicken with salt and pepper while it's still hot.

6. To make the aioli, in a medium bowl, combine mayonnaise, lemon juice, tomato paste, salt, garlic powder, and paprika. Stir to combine.

Copycat Culver's North Atlantic Cod Dinner

MAKES 4 SERVINGS

INGREDIENTS

- Nonstick cooking spray
- 3 Tbsp. olive oil
- 1/2 tsp. onion powder

- 1/2 tsp. garlic salt
- 1/2 tsp. black pepper
- 1 lb. sweet potatoes, cut into 1/2-inch-thick wedges
- 1/3 cup whole-wheat panko bread crumbs
- 1/2 tsp. dried thyme, crushed
- 1 lb. fresh or frozen cod fillets, about 1 inch thick, cut into serving-size pieces
- Lemon wedges or malt vinegar

HOW TO MAKE IT

1. Preheat oven to 425°F.

2. Line a 15×10-inch baking pan with foil; lightly coat with cooking spray. In a large bowl combine 1 Tbsp. of the oil, the onion powder, 1/4 tsp. of the garlic salt, and 1/4 tsp. of the pepper. Add potato wedges; toss to coat. Arrange in a single

layer on half of the prepared baking pan. Bake 15 minutes.

3. Meanwhile, in a small bowl combine bread crumbs, thyme, and the remaining 1/4 tsp. garlic salt and pepper. Add the remaining 2 Tbsp. oil; toss to combine.

4. Remove baking pan from oven. Carefully turn potatoes over. Place fish on the other half of the hot baking pan. Sprinkle crumb mixture onto fish; return to oven.

5. Bake about 10 minutes more or until potatoes are tender and starting to brown and fish flakes easily. Serve with lemon wedges or malt vinegar.

Copycat Panera Chicken Noodle Soup

MAKES 6 SERVINGS

INGREDIENTS

- 1 lb. boneless, skinless chicken breast
- 3 stalks of celery, sliced
- 3 carrots, peeled and sliced
- 1 medium onion, diced
- 2 garlic cloves, minced
- 1 tbsp thyme
- 1 tbsp rosemary
- 1 teaspoon salt
- 8 cups chicken stock
- 8 oz. egg noodles

HOW TO MAKE IT

1. Add the chicken, celery, carrots, onion, garlic cloves, thyme, and rosemary into the slow cooker.

2. Pour in the chicken stock.

3. Cook on high for 3-4 hours or low for 6-8 hours.

4. During the last 15 minutes, remove the chicken breast. Shred with a fork.

5. Add the chicken breast back in, as well as the egg noodles. Cook for the last 15 minutes.

Copycat TGI Friday's Spinach Artichoke Dip

SERVES 4

YOU'LL NEED

- 4 large whole-wheat pitas
- 1/2 Tbsp butter
- 1 onion, finely chopped
- 3 cloves garlic, finely chopped
- 1 jar (12 oz) artichoke hearts in water, drained and chopped
- 1 box (16 oz) chopped frozen spinach, thawed
- 1 can (4 oz) roasted green chiles, drained and chopped
- 2 Tbsp olive oil mayonnaise
- 2 Tbsp whipped cream cheese (Whipped cream cheese has air beaten into it, making it lighter and easier to spread.)
- Juice of 1 lemon
- Salt and black pepper to taste

HOW TO MAKE IT

1. Cut the pitas into 6 to 8 wedges each and separate the layers.

2. Spread on 2 baking sheets and bake at 400°F for 5 minutes or until crisp.

3. Heat the butter in a large skillet or sauté pan over medium heat.

4. Add the onion and garlic and cook for 5 minutes or until softened.

5. Add the artichokes, spinach, chiles, mayonnaise, cream cheese, and lemon juice.

6. Cook, stirring often, for 5 minutes or until hot. Season with salt and pepper.

7. Serve with the pita wedges.

Copycat P.F. Changs Shrimp Lo Mein

SERVES 4

YOU'LL NEED

- 12 oz lo mein noodles
- 1 tbsp peanut or vegetable oil
- 2 cloves garlic, minced
- 1 tbsp grated fresh ginger
- 4 scallions, whites and greens separated, chopped
- 4 oz shiitake mushrooms
- 2 medium carrots, cut into thin slices
- ½ red bell pepper, sliced
- ¾ lb medium shrimp, peeled and deveined
- 2 Tbsp oyster sauce
- 2 Tbsp low-sodium soy sauce

HOW TO MAKE IT

1. Prepare the noodles according to the package instructions.

2. In a wok or large skillet, heat the oil over high heat.

3. When the oil is lightly smoking, add the garlic, ginger, and scallion whites and stir-fry for 30 seconds, until lightly golden.

4. Add the mushrooms, carrots, and bell pepper, and continue cooking for 3 to 4 minutes, using a metal spatula to keep the vegetables in near-constant motion.

5. Toss in the shrimp and cook until just pink and slightly firm.

6. Add the cooked noodles, oyster sauce, and soy sauce to the pan.

7. Cook for 1 to 2 minutes more, until the sauce is thickened and covers the noodles in a light sheen.

8. Divide the mixture among 4 plates and garnish with the scallion greens.

Copycat Domino's Deluxe Pizza

SERVES 4

YOU'LL NEED

- 1 tsp olive oil
- 2 links Italian-style chicken sausage, casings removed
- 1 clove garlic, minced
- 1 bunch spinach, cleaned and stemmed
- Salt and black pepper to taste

- Pizza dough (Make your own, or buy 2 thin-crust store-bought pizza shells)
- 1 cup tomato sauce (make your own or buy a jar)
- 1 cup diced fresh mozzarella (or 1 cup shredded low-moisture mozzarella)
- 1/2 cup Peppadew peppers, or other bottled roasted peppers

HOW TO MAKE IT

1. Preheat the oven to 500°F. If you have a pizza stone, place it on the bottom rack of the oven.

2. Heat the olive oil in a large pan over medium heat.

3. Add the sausage and cook for about 3 minutes, until no longer pink.

4. Add the garlic and cook for 2 minutes more.

5. Add the spinach and cook, stirring, until wilted.

6. Drain any excess liquid gathered at the bottom pan. Season with salt and pepper.

7. On a lightly floured surface, stretch the dough into two 12" circles.

8. Working with one pizza at a time, place the pizza shell on a baking sheet, cover with a thin layer of tomato sauce, then top with half the mozzarella, spinach-sausage mixture, and peppers. (If using a stone, do this on a floured pizza peel, then slide the pizza onto the stone for baking.)

9. Bake for about 8 minutes, until the cheese is melted and bubbling and the crust is golden brown.

10. Cut each pie into 6 pieces. Repeat to make the second pizza.

Copycat Subway Chocolate Chip Cookies

MAKES ABOUT 12 COOKIES

YOU'LL NEED

- 8 tablespoons butter (1 stick), softened
- 1/2 cup packed brown sugar
- 1/2 cup granulated sugar
- 2 eggs
- 1 tsp vanilla extract
- 1/2 tsp baking soda

- 1/2 tsp salt (Salt teases out the flavors in any food it touches—even cookies. The crunchy crystals pair beautifully with the warm chocolate.)
- 2 cups flour
- 1/2 cup dark chocolate chips
- Flaky sea salt (optional)

HOW TO MAKE IT

1. Preheat the oven to 375°F.

2. In a mixing bowl, thoroughly mix the butter, brown sugar, and granulated sugar until creamy.

3. Stir in eggs and vanilla until well incorporated. Add the baking soda, salt, and flour, then mix until the dough comes together, being careful not to over-mix. Stir in the chocolate chips.

4. Drop the dough onto a baking sheet in balls about 3 tablespoons in size, leaving at least 3 inches between each.

5. Bake until the edges are golden and the middles are just barely set.

6. Remove from the sheet, sprinkle with a bit of sea salt (if using) and cool on a wire rack.

Copycat Charley's Philly Cheeseteaks

SERVES 4

YOU'LL NEED

1 lb skirt or flank steak

1/2 Tbsp canola or peanut oil, plus more if needed

1 large yellow onion, diced

1 medium green bell pepper, diced

2 cups sliced mushrooms

Salt and black pepper to taste

4 slices provolone

4 whole-wheat hoagie rolls, lightly toasted

HOW TO MAKE IT

1. Place the steak in the freezer for 20 minutes to firm up (this will help you slice it).

2. Use a very sharp knife to cut the thinnest strips possible from the beef.

3. Heat the oil in a large cast-iron skillet over medium heat.

4. Add the onions and cook for about 5 minutes, until soft and lightly browned.

5. Add the bell pepper and mushrooms and continue to cook for 5 to 7 minutes, until all of the vegetables are browned. Remove and reserve.

6. Swirl in enough oil to coat the bottom of the pan and add the sliced steak.

7. Season with salt and pepper right away, then use a spatula or tongs to keep the steak moving.

8. After the steak has browned on all sides (because it's thin, this will happen quickly—4 to 5 minutes).

9. Within the pan, divide the steak and veggie mixture into 4 equal piles and top each with a slice of provolone.

10. Continue cooking for about 1 minute, just until the provolone has melted.

11. Serve each pile on a hoagie roll.

Copycat Pei Wei Beef and Broccoli

MAKES 4-6 SERVINGS

INGREDIENTS

- 1 16 oz. flank steak, sliced thin
- 2 broccoli crowns, cut into florets (around 4-5 cups)
- 1/2 cup soy sauce
- 1 tablespoon rice vinegar
- 1 tablespoon brown sugar
- 2 teaspoons grated ginger
- 2 garlic cloves, minced
- 1 teaspoon Sriracha
- 1/2 teaspoon chili flakes
- 1 teaspoon honey
- 1 cup beef stock

- 1 tablespoon cornstarch

HOW TO MAKE IT

1. Add in the flank steak and broccoli florets to the slow cooker.

2. In a small bowl, whisk together the soy sauce, rice vinegar, brown sugar, sriracha, chili flakes, grated ginger, garlic, and honey.

3. Add in the sauce to the slow cooker, mix with the steak and broccoli.

4. Pour in the beef stock.

5. Turn the slow cooker on low for 2 hours.

6. During the last 30 minutes, mix together the cornstarch with 1/4 cup of water to make a slurry. Add the mixture to the crock-pot.

7. Serve on rice, and sprinkle sesame seeds, if desired.

Copycat California Pizza Kitchen BBQ Chicken Pizza

SERVES 4

YOU'LL NEED

For the pizza dough:

- 1 package instant yeast
- 1 cup hot water
- 1/2 tsp salt
- 1 Tbsp sugar or honey
- 1/2 Tbsp olive oil
- 21/2 cups flour, plus more for kneading and rolling

For the pizza:

- 3/4 cup barbecue sauce
- 1 1/2 cups shredded smoked gouda
- ½ red onion, thinly sliced
- ½ jalapeño pepper, thinly sliced
- 1 cup cooked chicken
- Fresh cilantro leaves

HOW TO MAKE IT

Make the Pizza Dough:

1. Combine yeast with the water, salt, and sugar or honey.

2. Allow to sit for 10 minutes while the hot water activates the yeast.

3. Stir in the olive oil and flour, using a wooden spoon to incorporate. When the dough is no longer sticky, place on a cutting board, cover with more flour, and knead for 5 minutes.

4. Return to the bowl, cover with plastic wrap, and let the dough rise at room temperature for at least 90 minutes.

5. Keeps covered in the refrigerator for up to 2 days.

...Now Make the Pizza:

1. Preheat the oven to 500°F. Place a pizza stone in the oven, if you have one.

2. Using your hands, a rolling pin, and enough flour to keep it from sticking, stretch the dough into two thin circles, 10" to 12" in diameter.

3. Spread each with a thin layer of barbecue sauce, then divide the gouda, onion, jalapeño, and chicken between the two.

4. If using a pizza stone, bake one pie at a time by carefully sliding the pizza (preferably with a pizza peel) onto the pizza stone; if you don't have a stone, cook the pizzas on a baking sheet.

5. The pizza is done when the crust is golden and the cheese is fully melted. Top with fresh cilantro, and cut into six or eight slices.

Copycat Chipotle Guacamole

SERVES 4

YOU'LL NEED

- 1/4 cup chopped cilantro
- 2 cloves garlic, minced
- Salt to taste
- 2 ripe avocados, pitted and peeled
- 1/4 cup minced onion

- 2 Tbsp minced jalapeño pepper
- Juice of 1 lemon
- 2 oz tortilla chips

HOW TO MAKE IT

1. Combine the cilantro and garlic on a cutting board and use the back of a chef's knife to work them into a fine paste; a pinch of coarse salt helps this process. (If you own a mortar and pestle, there's never been a better time to use it.)

2. Transfer the paste to a bowl and add the avocado.

3. Use a fork to mash the avocado into a mostly smooth—but still slightly chunky—purée.

4. Stir in the onion, jalapeño, lemon juice, and salt.

5. Serve with tortilla chips or warm corn tortillas.

Copycat Panda Express Orange Chicken

MAKES 4 SERVINGS

INGREDIENTS

- 1/2 tsp. orange zest
- 1/3 cup fresh orange juice
- 1/4 cup water
- 3 tbsp. honey
- 3 tbsp. reduced-sodium soy sauce
- 2 tbsp. rice vinegar
- 1 1/2 tbsp. cornstarch
- 2 cloves garlic, minced
- 1 tsp. grated fresh ginger
- 1/4 tsp. crushed red pepper

- 1 tbsp. canola oil
- 1 lb. skinless, boneless chicken breast, cut into bite-size pieces
- 1 cup bite-size strips red bell pepper
- 1 cup snow pea pods, halved diagonally
- 2 cups hot cooked brown rice
- 1/4 cup thinly sliced green onions
- 4 orange slices for serving (optional)

HOW TO MAKE IT

1. For sauce, in a small bowl stir together orange zest, orange juice, the water, honey, soy sauce, vinegar, cornstarch, garlic, ginger, and crushed red pepper.

2. In an extra-large nonstick skillet or wok heat oil over medium-high. Add chicken, pepper strips, and pea pods. Cook and stir about 5

minutes or until chicken is no longer pink. Stir sauce mixture and add to skillet. Cook and stir 1 to 2 minutes or until thickened and bubbly. Serve over rice; top with green onions and, if desired, orange slices and additional orange zest.

Copycat Wendy's Bacon Cheese Baked Potatoes

SERVES 4

YOU'LL NEED

- 2 medium russet potatoes
- Olive oil for coating the potatoes
- 4 strips bacon, cooked and crumbled (Cook the bacon for 15 minutes on a baking sheet alongside the potatoes.)

- 1/2 cup 2% milk
- 1 Tbsp butter
- 2 Tbsp Greek yogurt
- 1/2 cup chopped scallions (green parts only)
- 1/2 cup shredded sharp cheddar cheese
- Tabasco to taste
- Salt and black pepper to taste

HOW TO MAKE IT

1. Preheat the oven to 375°F. Prick the potatoes all over with a fork, then rub with a light layer of oil.

2. Place on the middle rack of the oven and bake for about 40 minutes, until tender all the way through. Increase the oven temperature to 450°F.

3. When the potatoes have cooled slightly, cut them in half lengthwise and carefully scoop out the flesh, being careful not to tear the skins.

4. Combine the potato flesh in a mixing bowl with the bacon, milk, butter, yogurt, scallions, about three-fourths of the cheese, Tabasco, and salt and pepper.

5. Mix thoroughly, then divide among the potato skins.

6. Top with the remaining cheese. Return to the oven and bake for 7 to 10 minutes, until browned on top.

Copycat Arby's Stuffed Jalapeño Bites

MAKES 4 SERVINGS

INGREDIENTS

- 10 jalapeño peppers, halved lengthwise and de-seeded
- 1/2 lb 80% lean ground beef
- 6 oz full-fat cream cheese
- 1 cup shredded cheddar cheese
- 4 slices cooked bacon
- 3/4 cup EPIC pork rinds

HOW TO MAKE IT

1. Preheat oven to 475°F. Line a baking sheet with foil.

2. Place the cream cheese and cheddar in a bowl of a sanding mixer fitted with a paddle attachment. Beat the cheeses together until they form a soft, creamy blend.

3. In a skillet over medium heat, cook the beef until brown all over, about 5 minutes.

4. Assemble the poppers by filling each with a spoonful of beef, and then covering with a generous amount of the cheese mix. Place on the baking sheet and bake for 10 minutes, until the filling is bubbling and has some brown spots. Feel free to broil to achieve the desired brownness.

5. While the peppers are baking, place cooked bacon and pork rinds in a food processor. Pulse until you get a crumbly texture. Once the poppers are done, sprinkle the topping over each popper. Serve immediately.

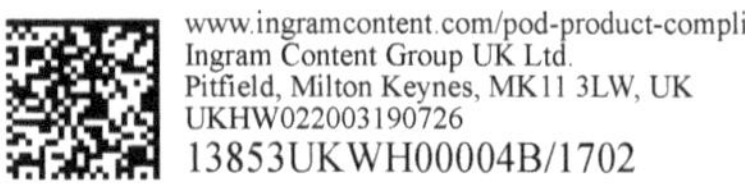
www.ingramcontent.com/pod-product-compliance
Ingram Content Group UK Ltd.
Pitfield, Milton Keynes, MK11 3LW, UK
UKHW022003190726
13853UKWH00004B/1702

9 798516 719875